Julio Cesar Romero Ramos
Wendy Johana Hernández Bedoya
Cristian Andrés Ramírez Hernández

Informal caregiver overload in patients with chronic diseases

Julio Cesar Romero Ramos
Wendy Johana Hernández Bedoya
Cristian Andrés Ramírez Hernández

Informal caregiver overload in patients with chronic diseases

in a primary health care provider, Monteria - Cordoba, 2023

ScienciaScripts

Imprint
Any brand names and product names mentioned in this book are subject to trademark, brand or patent protection and are trademarks or registered trademarks of their respective holders. The use of brand names, product names, common names, trade names, product descriptions etc. even without a particular marking in this work is in no way to be construed to mean that such names may be regarded as unrestricted in respect of trademark and brand protection legislation and could thus be used by anyone.

Cover image: www.ingimage.com

This book is a translation from the original published under ISBN 978-613-9-43403-9.

Publisher:
Sciencia Scripts
is a trademark of
Dodo Books Indian Ocean Ltd. and OmniScriptum S.R.L publishing group

120 High Road, East Finchley, London, N2 9ED, United Kingdom
Str. Armeneasca 28/1, office 1, Chisinau MD-2012, Republic of Moldova, Europe
Printed at: see last page
ISBN: 978-620-8-05066-5

Informal caregiver overload in patients with chronic diseases, in a primary health care provider, Montería - Córdoba, 2023.

Overload of the informal caregiver in patients with chronic diseases, in a primary health provider, Monteria - Córdoba, 2023.

Julio Cesar Romero Ramos *[1]

Master's Degree in Nursing - Universidad de Cartagena

Professor Universidad del Sinú Elías Bechara Zainum

julioromero@unisinu.edu.co

Wendy Johana Hernández Bedoya[2] **

Nurse Universidad del Sinú Elías Bechara Zainum

wendyjhernandez1@unisinu.edu.co

Montería. Córdoba. Colombia

Cristian Andrés Ramírez Hernández[3] ***

Nurse Universidad del Sinú Elías Bechara Zainum

cristianramirez@unisinu.edu.co

Montería. Córdoba. Colombia

TABLE OF CONTENTS

SUMMARY

Introduction: In recent years, with the progress of society in all areas, there has been an increase in life expectancy, and this has been accompanied by a change in the main causes of death and an increase in the prevalence of certain pathologies (chronic diseases and physical and/or mental disabilities), which condition a certain degree of dependence, with the elderly being the most affected population group.

Objectives: To identify informal caregiver overload in patients with chronic diseases in a primary health care provider, Montería - Córdoba, 2023 - 2.

Methodology: Quantitative study. It had a sample of 120 participants, which corresponds to the significant sample of the total population. After informed consent, the sociodemographic characteristics and overload of informal caregivers of patients with chronic diseases were identified. "Zarit Caregiver Burde Interview (Caregiver Burde Interview) Caregiver Overload Scale". Descriptive statistical analysis allowed the data to be represented in frequencies and percentages.

Results: 120 informal caregivers participated: 77% were women and 23% were men. Sixty-nine percent were from urban areas, 31% from rural areas. Education: high school (48.2%) or technical/higher education (32.5%). Marital status: single 36.6%, married 31.8%, common-law 26.6%. Housewives 42.5%, self-employed 27.5%, employed 22.5%. Stratum I (80%), stratum II 20%. Caring for children (58.3%) Spouse 15%. Hours of caregiving 6-12 hours 52.5%. 12 - 18 hours 25.8%. At the overall level of informal caregiver overload, is the absence of overload with 66%, followed by light overload with 19%, and 15% intense overload.

Conclusion: The results made it possible to meet the study objectives and identify a positive correlation between caregiving competencies and informal caregiver overload, which can be interpreted as "the higher the caregiving competencies, the lower the level of overload". These findings show that informal caregivers and primary health care providers have various competencies and skills to optimally exercise their roles as caregivers and health care providers and therefore have the ability to cope with situations of overload.

The functional dependence of the chronic patient on his or her caregiver was established by the number of hours spent by the informal caregiver in his or her care, with a functional dependence ratio of 79%.

Keywords: Burden, Overload, Informal caregiver, Chronic diseases, Functional dependency (Source: DsSc)

INTRODUCTION

The World Health Organization WHO 2021 (1), reported statistics in October 2021, that between 2020 and 2030, the number of inhabitants of the planet over 60 years of age will increase 34%, in this same order of ideas, points out that currently, people live longer than before, which has contributed to increase conservation and longevity; by the year 2030, one out of every six people in the world will be 60 years old or older. With the above, it is important to note that at the same rate that people increase their years of life, they can also present various pathologies.
Pardo Y, Chaparro L, Carreño S 2022 (2), affirm that in this course of life, chronic non-communicable diseases appear that can generate a certain degree of disability and dependence, which will cause most of the long-lived to need constant accompaniment, someone to assist them either in the care of their illness or to help them perform the basic activities of daily life that they cannot perform on their own.

Caring for a dependent loved one is a stressful condition, the psychological, physical and mental consequences of which are diverse and have been investigated. Numerous studies have demonstrated the negative impact of the caregiver experience on the mental health of caregivers, highlighting the development of symptoms of anxiety and depression, irritability and stress-related physical problems, among other problems. These effects have been found in caregivers where their loved ones suffer from a cone disease, as discussed by Guato P, Mendoza S 2022 (3).

Being a caregiver of a frail person or dependent adult is a great challenge, as expressed by Fernández B, Herrera S 2020(4), when stating that this role commonly harms the physical health and well-being of caregivers. Several authors agree that, given the environment of illness and dependence of a person, whoever is responsible for exercising the role of caregiver is subjected to a level of burden, which will have a negative impact on their health, this performance can trigger psychological disorders such as anxiety and depression. Cardenas D 2022 (5).

In this research it is important to mention that the most widely used caregiver assessment instrument in the Spanish language is the Zarit Care Burden Perception Interview. This questionnaire, which consists of 22 items, emerged mainly to evaluate caregivers of people with dementia, determines the burden experienced by the caregiver through a global score, thus presenting a unidimensional conception despite containing items that refer to different aspects of the burden. It should be noted that caregiver burden is not limited only to informal caregivers, which has allowed the instrument to measure formal caregiver burden in direct care nursing staff.

The elaboration and execution of this research is relevant, since the results will help to visualize the situation of informal caregivers, the effects and the level of burden they experience. The need for accompaniment of caregivers, either by the state or health institutions and even more important, the different professionals of the interdisciplinary health teams, will become evident. Abdellatif O 2022 (6).

2. PROBLEM STATEMENT

An informal caregiver is a person who does not belong to the health area and is responsible for the task of caring for sick, disabled or elderly people who are unable to take care of themselves to carry out activities of daily living (cleaning, feeding, mobility, dressing, etc.), administer treatment or go to the health services. Informal caregivers are the main people who are in charge of the care of chronic patients and provide them with support within their environment without receiving any type of remuneration. Martínez S 2020 (7).

When we talk about chronic patients, we refer to those people who have long-term conditions, but with a generally slow progression as a result of this, we can see that it is a public health problem for today and also a major cause of death for people with this condition, which would demand greater attention from caregivers to these patients, making them more vulnerable to present illness and affect their quality of life. In addition, generally those who exercise the role of caregivers are members of the nuclear family; they are attentive to their integrity, to provide the basic care that people with decreased or loss of functionality require. When a person requires the care of another person, new contexts or situations are generated that induce important changes within the family dynamics and structure, as well as in the roles and even in the behavior patterns of its members, according to Murillo D, Fernández E, Velasco E 2019 (8). The aforementioned changes, according to Celeiro T 2019 (9), can lead to crises that jeopardize family stability, which would affect the entire family unit, but primarily the primary caregiver, who is the family member who bears most of the physical and emotional excess of the care provided to the affected person.

In the same vein, they reflect and establish that caregiver burnout involves various spheres: physical health, mental health, absence of time or space, very limited time to perform their activities, social withdrawal, detriment to the economic situation and, in general, impairment of the quality of life, which is called caregiver syndrome, as expressed by Ulloa O 2019 (10).

Regarding this syndrome, Menéndez T 2019 (11), expresses that those who manage to suffer from it, are frequently subjected to stressful circumstances, which could generate risks, by exhausting the caregiver's capacities and likewise affecting physical health and mood. For the correct management of these situations, it is important to have an excellent relationship within the health team and the family, constantly educating the mechanisms and protection strategies for the integral health of the caregiver.

However, the person in charge of ensuring this care can also face or assume positions of resilience, where he/she seeks to adapt to different situations, many of these positions may be loving and supportive relationships within and outside the family, recreational spaces, physical rest, among others. A relationship that radiates love and trust provides role models, encouragement and confidence, which help to demonstrate human resilience. Aguinaga S 2022 (12).

It is important to remember that on many occasions the caregiver's health takes second place, focusing specifically on the person in his or her care, i.e., all actions are focused on the caregiver. Therefore, it is evident that the situation of dependence and vulnerability of the patient causes little interest, directly or indirectly, in the caregiver's health, and this should be addressed as a priority, due to the importance it implies for the caregiver and the person under his or her care. González C 2022 (13).

Therefore, it is necessary to always keep in mind that the care offered by the health care team must intervene holistically and integrally in the patient and thus contribute to the reduction of the overload that this person may be experiencing.

According to WHO statistics, more than 40 million people die annually from Chronic non-communicable diseases and the leading causes of death are cardiovascular diseases (17.7 million each year), followed by cancer (8.8 million), respiratory diseases (3.9 million) and diabetes (1.6 million). These four groups of conditions are responsible for more than 80% of all premature deaths from chronic noncommunicable disease NCDs. Serra M 2020 (14).

These diseases generate certain complications, which increase in the course of life in old age, generating certain anatomical and physiological changes that diminish the person's ability to perform the instrumental activities of daily living, which makes it necessary to have a person to support the daily exercise of this person, and it is where the family takes an important and significant role or a person who keeps affection and sacrifice Noa Y 2021 (15).

Generally, those who exercise the role of caregivers are members of the family nucleus; they are attentive to their integrity, to provide the basic care that people with diminished or loss of functionality require. When a person requires the care of another person, new contexts or situations are generated that induce important changes within the family dynamics and structure, as well as in the roles and even in the behavior patterns of its members, according to Arias C 2019 (16). The aforementioned changes, as stated by Hernández J 2022 (17), can lead to crises that jeopardize family stability, which would affect the entire family unit, but primarily the primary caregiver, who is the family member who bears most of the physical and emotional excess of the care provided to the affected person.

In the same vein, they reflect and establish that caregiver burnout involves various spheres: physical health, mental health, absence of time or space, very limited time to perform their activities, social withdrawal, detriment to the economic situation and, in general, impairment of the quality of life, which is called caregiver syndrome Moreno A 2020 (18).

Regarding this syndrome, Menéndez T 2019 (19), expresses that those who manage to suffer from it, are frequently subjected to stressful circumstances, which could generate risks, by exhausting the caregiver's capacities and likewise affecting physical health and mood. For the correct management of these situations, it is important to have an excellent relationship within the health team and the family, constantly educating the mechanisms and protection strategies for the integral health of the caregiver.

However, the person in charge of ensuring this care can also face or assume positions of resilience, where he/she seeks to adapt to different situations, many of these positions may be loving and supportive relationships within and outside the family, recreational spaces, physical rest, among others. A relationship that radiates love and trust provides role models, encouragement and confidence, which help to demonstrate human resilience. Cardenas C 2021 (20)

It is important to remember that on many occasions the caregiver's health takes second place, focusing specifically on the person in his or her care, i.e., all actions are focused on the caregiver. Therefore, it is clear that the situation of dependence and vulnerability of the patient causes little interest, directly or indirectly, in the caregiver's health, and this should be addressed as a priority, due to the importance it implies for the caregiver and the person under his or her care. Rabelo A 2022 (21).

Therefore, it is necessary to always keep in mind that the care offered by the health care team must intervene holistically and integrally in the patient and thus contribute to the reduction of the overload that this person may be experiencing.

In this order of ideas, it is convenient to carry out a study on the meaning of the caregiver's burden, which helps to understand the difficulties that these caregivers must face, but also to inquire about those methods of strengthening that each caregiver can develop. Currently, there is evidence of an academic increase in the number of research studies on the physical, mental and social health of caregivers, especially informal caregivers, and this should take into consideration the vulnerability of this significant group. In addition, it will serve as a contribution to increase the understanding, sensitivity, respect and commitment that we as students and as teachers should have with informal caregivers, as they are very much forgotten nowadays.

2.1 Research Question:

What is the overload of the informal caregiver in patients with chronic diseases in a primary health care provider, Montería - Córdoba 2023?

3. OBJECTIVES

3.1 General:

To identify informal caregiver overload in patients with chronic diseases in a primary health care provider, Montería - córdoba, 2023.

3.2 Specific:

- To identify the sociodemographic characteristics of the informal caregiver of patients with chronic diseases Montería Córdoba 2023.
- To determine informal caregiver overload in patients with chronic diseases in a primary health care provider in Montería Córdoba 2023.
- To establish a statistical association between the number of hours spent by informal caregivers caring for their family member and their functional dependence.
- To establish statistical association between sociodemographic characteristics and level of overload of informal caregivers of patients with diseases.

4. JUSTIFICATION

As reported by the National Administrative Department of Statistics DANE 2022 (22), "the leading cause of death was ischemic heart disease, which registered 41,783 deaths; second place went to cerebrovascular diseases, which accounted for 14,390; and third place to chronic respiratory diseases, which claimed 12,857".

Chronic diseases represent a high prevalence and incidence in our country that in advanced complications require special support, being vital the support of a caregiver who is responsible for the patient's condition. At present, caregiver overload Garcia Y 2022 (23), says that it is a fairly common problem in our society which has not shown interest, but it is important to treat it due to the health consequences that the caregiver and the cared subject may have in their development. For this reason, the following research work will be carried out in order to know the degree of disability of the elderly and to know the level of overload of the main caregivers of the population under study.

On the other hand, to date there is no research at the local level in Cordoba-Montería on the level of overload of the main caregivers of patients with chronic dependent diseases. In-depth research could help prevent psychological and social problems in caregivers as well as help promote situational and personal characteristics that allow caregivers to have a better quality of life, thus avoiding that the main caregiver ends up becoming in the future a caregiver for another sick person.

The elaboration of the mentioned project is justified firstly by the contribution of scientific and statistical studies related to the real health problems identified in the community, which will allow us to inform the subjects of study, their condition in connection with the real pathology and how to treat it in the appropriate way in early stages in order to prevent complications in the medium and long term. This will also contribute to the caregiver's quality of life and thus to his or her task of caring for the cared-for subject.

In conclusion, the study will seek a result to the identified problems, for this reason the results obtained will serve to adopt preventive measures that will be taught by health professionals through education and health promotion, as well as to promote self-care to avoid health consequences, emphasizing that to care we must first learn to take care of ourselves; all this in order to avoid both a caregiver burden syndrome and the exacerbation of the state of dependence of the elderly.

Social Significance: The results of this research will contribute to improve the way in which caregivers assume their self-care in order to provide quality care. On the other hand, it will allow to make some recommendations regarding caregivers in order to strengthen their management within the health system. the results will inform society about the repercussions in the daily life of caregivers of independent older adults, thus generating a critical and reflective look on this current phenomenon, In addition to this, it will also allow the nursing professional to elaborate new tools and strategies that will help to elaborate a public health plan benefiting the caregiver and health professionals, thus reducing the increase of the consequences that this problem brings with it. Cruz L 2022 (24)

Theoretical Significance: The theoretical contribution of this research seeks to provide greater knowledge regarding the complications that bring with them the performance of a caregiver of a patient with a chronic disease, focusing not only on chronic patient or not, but also on the caregiver as a fundamental unit for the recovery of his or her health. In addition to this, it was concluded that there are gaps at the theoretical level, we can say that it has been little studied at the departmental level, besides there is a shortage of study regarding the ongoing phenomenon at the national level.

Therefore, the current research will be oriented based on the theory of Henderson V (25) with the theory of care, which is based on the person's ability to maintain independence. This theory focuses on 14 important theoretical needs that all humans have, each of which constitutes the integrating element of physical, social, psychological and spiritual aspects. This role is fundamental to carry out the achievement of our object of study giving us the advantage of knowing possible solutions to the problems that currently occur. Doicela R 2020 (26).

Disciplinary Significance: The results obtained will allow us to recognize which are the most relevant reasons that predispose in the daily life of the affected people, this will allow us to elaborate promotion and prevention nursing activities directed to those risk factors that compromise the quality of life of this population.

In addition, knowledge based on scientific evidence will be obtained in order to improve the Nursing Care Process (PAE) oriented to know the factors causing the complications associated with this problem, thus promoting the prevention and care of patients in the department of Córdoba. Elso R (27)

5. CONCEPTUAL FRAMEWORK

5.1 Chronic Disease.

A chronic disease is a long-term health condition that generally has no cure and tends to persist for prolonged periods or even the patient's entire life. Unlike acute diseases that have a rapid onset and limited duration, chronic diseases are characterized by slower development and gradual progression. These diseases can have a variety of causes, including genetic, environmental, lifestyle and other unknown factors.

Chronic diseases encompass a wide variety of conditions, such as type 2 diabetes, cardiovascular diseases (such as high blood pressure and coronary heart disease), chronic lung diseases (such as asthma and chronic obstructive pulmonary disease - COPD), autoimmune diseases (such as rheumatoid arthritis and lupus), chronic neurological diseases (such as Parkinson's disease and multiple sclerosis), among others.

A common characteristic of chronic diseases is that, although they cannot be completely cured, they can be controlled and managed with medical treatments, therapies and lifestyle changes. Proper management of these diseases usually involves taking regular medication, continuous medical follow-up, adopting a balanced diet, exercising, avoiding smoking and excessive alcohol consumption, and stress management.

Chronic diseases can have a significant impact on a patient's quality of life and can also affect their ability to carry out daily activities, work and participate in social activities. In addition, they can increase the risk of serious complications and long-term disability. Arias E 2019 (28).

Family Caregiver

Refers to a person seeking medical or health care due to the presence of symptoms, illnesses, injuries or health conditions that require diagnosis, treatment and follow-up by health professionals. Patients may go to hospitals, clinics, doctors' offices or care centers to receive care from doctors, nurses, specialists and other healthcare professionals who are engaged in providing health and wellness services. The relationship between patient and healthcare professional is critical, involving effective communication, empathy, respect and trust to ensure proper care and optimal recovery.

The patient care process begins with a medical history, where information is gathered about the patient's symptoms, medical history, medications and lifestyle habits. From this information, a physical examination is performed and, in many cases, diagnostic tests are ordered to identify the underlying cause of the symptoms. Once a diagnosis is established, the healthcare professional and patient work together to develop a personalized treatment plan that may include medications, therapies, surgical interventions or other medical procedures.

In addition to addressing the specific disease or condition, patient care also focuses on promoting prevention and self-care to improve quality of life and prevent future complications. Patient education about their condition is encouraged and guidance is provided to make informed decisions about their health.

Patient care involves not only medical aspects, but also emotional and psychological aspects. Health professionals should consider the emotional needs of the patient and provide support throughout the treatment process, as the emotional impact of the disease can be significant. Sierra L 2019 (29).

5.3 Caregiver.

A caregiver is a person who assumes responsibility for providing support, assistance and care to another individual who needs help due to illness, disability, old age or other condition that limits his or her ability to perform daily activities independently. Caregivers may be family members, friends, or hired professionals who devote their time and effort to ensure the well-being and safety of the individual they care for.

The caregiver's work can be varied and demanding, involving tasks such as helping with personal grooming, feeding, mobility, administering medications, coordinating medical appointments and constant supervision. In addition to practical tasks, caregivers also provide emotional and social support, as the relationship with the person they care for can be close and meaningful.

Being a caregiver can have a significant impact on the caregiver's own life. They can experience considerable physical and emotional strain due to the dedication and responsibility that comes with constantly caring for another person. Stress, exhaustion and feelings of isolation are common challenges faced by caregivers, highlighting the importance of caregivers receiving support and attention as well.

In many cases, the caregiving role also involves making difficult decisions, such as managing medical treatments or planning for long-term care. The need to balance the demands of caregiving with other aspects of life, such as work and one's own family responsibilities, can be overwhelming.

It is essential to recognize the invaluable work that caregivers provide to society and to ensure that they have access to resources and services that enable them to care for both themselves and their loved ones adequately. Warrior D 2023 (30).

5.4 Patient's caregiver.

A patient caregiver is a person who provides care and support to a patient who has an illness or disability, either at home or in another health care setting. Patient caregivers may be family members, friends, or professional health care providers: the role of the patient caregiver is essential in the health care process, as they can provide physical, emotional, and social assistance to the patient. This includes tasks such as assisting with personal hygiene, administering medications, and monitoring the patient's diet, among others. The patient's caregivers can also act as advocates for the patient, communicating their needs and concerns to healthcare providers and ensuring that they receive appropriate care. Often, the role of the patient's caregiver can be very stressful and overwhelming, and adequate support is required to ensure their well-being and ability to provide adequate patient care. Aguado E 2019 (31).

5.5 Family Caregiver

A family caregiver is a person who assumes the responsibility of providing unpaid care to a dependent family member. These individuals perform a variety of tasks, including helping with activities of daily living, monitoring medical treatment, assisting with mobility, feeding and grooming, and handling administrative procedures, among others.

Family caregivers may be children, spouses, siblings or other close relatives of the patient, and often serve in this role on a long-term, ongoing basis. While a valuable and necessary task, caring for an ill or dependent family member can create a number of physical, emotional, and financial challenges for the caregiver. Esquivel N 2021 (32) .

5.6 Functional dependence.

The functional status is measured through the result of developing basic activities of daily living, when the person lacks the ability to perform them, it is recognized as functional dependence, i.e., this is the one in which there is an absence of capacity or decrease of this, to perform some activity without requiring assistance. Baracaldo H 2019 (33).

5.7 Quality of life.

Defined as "an individual's perception of his or her place in life, in the context of the culture and value system in which he or she lives, and in relation to his or her goals, expectations, standards and concerns".

There are several scales and tools used to measure and assess quality of life, both in general populations and in specific groups such as patients with chronic diseases or disabilities. These tools take into account different aspects of quality of life, such as physical and mental health, life satisfaction, emotional and social well-being, among others. Salinas A 2022 (34)

5.8 Caregiver care conditions

Caregiver caregiving conditions refer to factors that may affect the quality of life, health, and emotional well-being of family caregivers who assume the responsibility of caring for a dependent family member. These conditions include:

Emotional overload: Caring for a family member can be emotionally demanding, which can cause stress, anxiety, depression and emotional exhaustion.

Physical overload: Caregivers may experience fatigue, muscle aches, sleep problems and other physical problems related to ongoing caregiving.

Lack of social support: Lack of support and understanding from friends, family and the community can leave the caregiver feeling isolated and discouraged.

Financial problems: Caring for a dependent family member can generate significant financial costs, which can jeopardize the caregiver's financial stability.

Lack of personal time: Caregivers often have little time to devote to their own needs and activities, which can affect their quality of life and emotional well-being. In order for family caregivers to provide effective and healthy care for their loved ones, it is important that they receive the support and resources needed to manage these caregiving conditions. Zuluaga M 2021 (35)

5.9 Sole Caregiver

The term "sole caregiver" refers to the person who assumes primary responsibility for caring for a dependent family member, and who does not have the support or assistance of other family members or caregivers. This type of caregiver faces a unique set of challenges, such as social isolation, emotional and physical overload, and lack of time to attend to his or her own needs.

Sole caregivers may experience a higher level of stress and health problems compared to those who have the support of other caregivers or family members. In addition, lack of support may also increase the caregiver's risk of experiencing depression, anxiety, and other mental health problems. It is important to recognize that sole caregiving is not always a choice, and that some caregivers may find themselves in this situation due to the lack of resources or support available in their community. As such, it is important that health care providers and health care professionals provide adequate support and resources to ensure that sole caregivers can provide the best possible care for their loved ones without sacrificing their own health and well-being. Rivera M 2021 (36).

5.1.1 Loading

The term "burden" is commonly used to describe the emotional and physical impact that caring for a dependent family member can have on a caregiver's life. Burden can include a variety of factors, such as stress, anxiety, depression, physical overload, and lack of time to attend to the caregiver's own needs.

Caregiving burden can affect both the caregiver and the patient and can have long-term consequences. Burden can negatively affect the caregiver's physical and emotional health, which can lead to long-term health problems such as chronic illness, depression and anxiety. In addition, it can also affect the quality of care provided to the patient, which can have negative consequences on the patient's health and well-being.

It is important to recognize the burden caregiving can have on a caregiver's life and provide appropriate support to help reduce the burden and improve the caregiver's and patient's quality of life. Martinez L 2019 (37).

5.1.2 Caregiver Burden.

Caregiver burden, also known as caregiver burden or family caregiver burden, refers to the set of physical, emotional and financial responsibilities that fall on the caregiver of a loved one with an illness, disability or chronic health condition. This burden can significantly affect the caregiver's quality of life and impact the caregiver's physical and emotional health.

Caregiver burden can manifest itself in a variety of ways. Physically, the caregiver may experience increased fatigue and exhaustion due to ongoing caregiving tasks, such as mobilizing the patient, assisting with personal hygiene, and administering medications. In addition, caregivers often have to balance their caregiving responsibilities with their own work and family obligations, which can create an overload on their time and energy.

Emotionally, caregivers may face elevated levels of stress, anxiety and depression. Constant concern for the patient's health and well-being, as well as uncertainty about the future, can generate significant emotional strain. In addition, some caregivers may feel isolated and lacking in social support, as the dedication to caregiving responsibilities may limit their participation in social and recreational activities.

Financial burden is also a major concern for many caregivers. Care-related expenses such as medications, medical treatments, specialized equipment and home care services can be costly and add additional strain on the caregiver's finances.

It is critical to recognize the importance of supporting caregivers and providing them with resources to help them cope more effectively with the burden of caregiving. Access to respite programs, support groups, home care services, and counseling can be helpful in easing the burden and improving caregiver well-being. Mora B 2020 (38).

5.1.3 Caregiver overload.

Caregiver overload, also known as caregiving overload or family caregiver overload, refers to a condition in which the person assuming caregiving responsibility for a loved one experiences an overwhelming level of physical, emotional, and psychological demands related to caregiving. This overload can arise when the caregiver is faced with an excessive burden of responsibilities and does not have sufficient support or resources to cope with the demands of caregiving.

From the physical point of view, caregiver overload may manifest itself in physical exhaustion due to constant and demanding caregiving tasks. The caregiver may have to assist with the patient's daily activities, such as grooming, mobilization or feeding, which may require considerable physical exertion. Lack of time for adequate rest and self-care can lead to deterioration of the caregiver's physical health.

Emotionally, caregiver overload can lead to high levels of stress, anxiety and depression. Constant concern for the patient's well-being, especially if the patient has a serious medical condition, can cause great emotional toll. In addition, caregivers often experience feelings of guilt, frustration, or helplessness when faced with difficulties in providing needed care.

Caregiver overload can also have an impact on the caregiver's social life. The time and energy devoted to caregiving can limit participation in social and recreational activities, which can lead to isolation and lack of social support.

It is important to note that caregiver overload affects not only the caregiver but also the patient. When the caregiver is overburdened, he or she may not be able to provide quality care to the patient, which can negatively affect the health and well-being of the loved one receiving care.

To address caregiver overload, it is essential to provide adequate support and resources. Respite programs, access to home care services, support groups, and counseling can help alleviate caregiver burden and improve overall well-being. Soriano L 2022 (39).

5.1.4 Overload Ratings

Overload ratings are a way of measuring the subjective burden experienced by a family caregiver in relation to caring for a dependent family member.

Overload ratings are used to assess the intensity and impact of the emotional, social and physical burden that a caregiver may experience.

The most commonly used overload rating scale is the Zarit Caregiver Overload Scale (ZBI), which assesses subjective burden in several domains, such as caregiver physical and emotional health, relationship with the patient, and time spent caregiving. The Zarit scale is a useful tool for identifying caregivers who may be at greater risk of experiencing overload and who may require additional support.

Degrees of overload can range from mild to severe levels, and can have a significant impact on caregiver and patient quality of life. It is important to recognize the degrees of overload experienced by caregivers and provide appropriate support to help reduce burden and improve caregiver and patient quality of life. Navarro M 2019 (40)

5.1.5 Number of hours of assistance required daily for care.

The number of hours of assistance a patient requires daily for care is a critical aspect that can vary significantly depending on the patient's health condition and level of dependency. This measure is important for assessing the intensity of care a person needs and for planning the appropriate resources and support to meet his or her needs.

The number of hours of assistance needed can range from a few hours a day for those who need assistance with specific tasks, to full-time care for patients with more complex care needs. Some of the care activities that may require assistance include personal grooming, medication administration, mobilization, feeding, transportation and emotional support.

The number of hours of care needed may also change over time due to the evolution of the patient's health condition. Some illnesses may progress, requiring an increase in the amount of care and assistance needed, while in other cases, with an improvement in the patient's health, the hours of care may decrease.

In addition, it is important to consider the role of caregivers and family members in providing care. Care may be provided by family members, friends, health care professionals, or contracted caregivers. Depending on the availability and capacity of caregivers, the number of hours of care needed may vary.

Carefully assessing a patient's care needs is essential to ensure that he or she receives appropriate care and that caregivers are supported in fulfilling this important task. A proper assessment will allow resources to be planned and allocated more effectively, providing quality care and improving the quality of life of both the patient and his or her caregivers. Garcia A 2019 (41).

5.1.6 Health.

Health is a complete state of physical, mental and social well-being, and not merely the absence of disease or infirmity. It is a dynamic and multifaceted state that implies an optimal balance between body, mind and the social environment in which a person lives.

From a physical standpoint, health refers to the condition of the body and its ability to function properly. This includes aspects such as having a strong immune system, good cardiovascular and respiratory function, adequate nutrition, and the ability to perform daily activities without significant difficulties.

From a mental point of view, health implies psychological, emotional and cognitive well-being. This includes having a positive and resilient attitude towards life's challenges, maintaining good mental and emotional health, and having the ability to cope effectively with stress and difficulties. In addition, health is also closely related to the social environment in which a person lives. This includes having access to quality health care services, a safe and clean environment, a strong social support network, and opportunities to participate in social and community activities.

Health promotion involves promoting healthy habits and lifestyles that contribute to improving and maintaining well-being in all its dimensions. This includes a balanced and nutritious diet, regular physical exercise, avoiding smoking and excessive alcohol consumption, getting adequate sleep, and managing stress in a positive way.

Disease prevention and early detection of health problems are also important components of health. Regular medical checkups, vaccinations and access to timely medical care help maintain health and prevent serious complications. It is important to recognize that health is a valuable resource that enables people to reach their full potential and participate fully in society. Moreover, health is a fundamental human right and a shared responsibility of individuals, communities, and governments to ensure optimal conditions of well-being for all. Hurtado D 2021 (42).

5.1.7 Social security system.

The social security system is an institutional structure designed and managed by the State for the purpose of protecting the population against various social and economic risks that may affect their welfare and quality of life. This system is based on principles of solidarity, equity and social justice, seeking to ensure that all people have access to essential services and benefits, regardless of their economic capacity or employment status.

The social security system usually encompasses different areas of protection and is organized into different branches, each oriented to meet specific needs of the population. The main branches of the social security system include:

Social security in health: Guarantees access to health care services, treatments and medicines necessary to maintain and improve people's health. This branch seeks to protect the population against disease and promote disease prevention and health promotion.

Social security pensions: Provides economic income to workers in their retirement or retirement stage, ensuring that they can maintain an adequate and dignified standard of living after their working life.

Social security for occupational risks: Protects workers against accidents or illnesses related to their employment, providing economic, medical and rehabilitation assistance to facilitate their recovery and reintegration to work.

Unemployment social security: Provides temporary financial support to people who have lost their jobs, helping them to cover their basic needs while they look for a new job opportunity.

Social security for maternity and childhood: Seeks to protect pregnant women and mothers, as well as children, through benefits and services that contribute to their well-being during this vital stage.

The financing of the social security system comes from different sources, including contributions from employers and workers, public funds, specific taxes and other sources of financing established by the legislation of each country. SDS 2023 (43).

5.1.8 Cancer

Cancer is a complex and devastating disease that affects millions of people worldwide. It is a group of diseases characterized by the uncontrolled and abnormal growth of cells in the body, resulting in the formation of tumors or masses of malignant tissue. These cancerous cells can invade nearby tissues and spread to other parts of the body through the lymphatic system or bloodstream, in a process known as metastasis.

Cancer can develop in virtually any part of the body and can affect people of all ages. There are numerous types of cancer, classified according to the organ or tissue in which they originate. Some of the most common types include lung cancer, breast cancer, prostate cancer, colon cancer, skin cancer, pancreatic cancer and many others.

The exact causes of cancer are multifactorial and in many cases not fully understood. However, it is known that certain factors can increase the risk of developing cancer, such as smoking, excessive alcohol consumption, unhealthy diet, exposure to chemicals and radiation, obesity and hereditary genetic factors.

Early diagnosis is critical to the successful treatment of cancer. Cancer symptoms can vary widely depending on the type and stage of the disease, but may include unexplained weight loss, persistent fatigue, skin changes, difficulty swallowing, abnormal bleeding and other symptoms specific to each type of cancer.

Cancer treatment depends on the type and stage of the disease, as well as the individual characteristics of the patient.

The emotional and psychological impact of cancer on patients and their families should not be underestimated. A cancer diagnosis can cause great anxiety, fear and emotional stress. It is essential to provide comprehensive and compassionate support to patients and their loved ones throughout the treatment and recovery process. Tinoco A 2019 (44).

5.1.9 Heart disease

Heart disease is a broad term that encompasses a group of diseases and disorders that affect the heart and circulatory system. These conditions can vary in severity and symptoms, but they all have in common the fact that they interfere with the proper functioning of the heart, the organ responsible for pumping blood and distributing oxygen and nutrients throughout the body.

One of the most common forms of heart disease is coronary heart disease, also known as coronary artery disease. This disease is characterized by the accumulation of deposits of fat, cholesterol and other substances in the coronary arteries that supply blood to the heart. Over time, these accumulations form plaques that can narrow or partially or completely block the arteries, reducing blood flow to the heart. This can lead to angina pectoris (chest pain) or, in the case of total blockage, a myocardial infarction or heart attack.

Another common form of heart disease is heart failure, which occurs when the heart cannot pump enough blood to meet the body's demands. Heart failure can be caused by a variety of factors, such as damage to the heart muscle due to a previous heart attack, uncontrolled high blood pressure, valve disease, or heart muscle disease.

Treatment of heart disease depends on the type and severity of the disease, but may include lifestyle changes, such as quitting smoking, eating a healthy diet, and exercising regularly. Medications may also be used to control blood pressure, lower cholesterol, stabilize heart rhythm or improve heart function. In more severe cases, medical procedures, such as coronary angioplasty or coronary bypass surgery, may be necessary to restore adequate blood flow to the heart.

Prevention of heart disease is fundamental and is based on the adoption of healthy lifestyle habits, control of risk factors, and early detection and treatment of underlying conditions. Education about the importance of leading a healthy lifestyle and access to regular medical care are key components in the prevention and management of heart disease. Ruperti J 2020 (45).

5.2.1 Cardiovascular accident

A cerebrovascular accident (CVA), also known as an ictus or stroke, occurs when blood flow to the brain is interrupted, either by blockage of a blood vessel or by its rupture. This interruption of blood flow can cause brain damage and have serious consequences for the health and quality of life of the person affected.

Stroke as "a brain injury caused by an interruption of the blood supply to the brain. An ischemic stroke occurs when an artery supplying blood to the brain is blocked by a blood clot. A hemorrhagic stroke occurs when a cerebral artery ruptures and bleeding occurs in the brain."

Risk factors for stroke include high blood pressure, diabetes, obesity, advanced age, smoking and excessive alcohol consumption. Treatment of stroke depends on the type and severity of the brain injury, and may include medication, occupational therapy, and physical therapy. Canchos M 2019 (46).

5.2.2 Arthritis

Arthritis is a chronic inflammatory disease affecting the joints of the human body. It is characterized by pain, swelling, stiffness and loss of motion in the affected joints. There are more than 100 different types of arthritis, the most common forms being osteoarthritis and rheumatoid arthritis.

Osteoarthritis is the most common form of arthritis, which occurs when the protective cartilage covering the joints wears down over time, which can cause pain and stiffness. Rheumatoid arthritis, on the other hand, is an autoimmune disease in which the immune system attacks the joints themselves, causing inflammation and pain.

In addition to affecting the joints, arthritis can have other effects on the body, such as fatigue, fever and weight loss. It can also cause permanent joint damage, which can limit a person's ability to perform daily activities.

The diagnosis of arthritis is based on the symptoms that the person presents, as well as on the results of medical tests, such as blood tests and X-rays. Urbina Y 2020 (47).

6. THEORETICAL FRAMEWORK

According to the World Health Organization WHO 2022 (48), chronic diseases are defined as those ailments that have a prolonged permanence in the human body with a generally slow progression until they exhaust the body, and are the result of a combination of genetics, physiological, environmental and behavioral factors of the population that suffers from them.

There are multiple causes and disabilities that are related to the progress of a dependency, as expressed by Lorca M 2021 (49), in his research, the aging of the population as an external cause, in addition to malnutrition, child neglect, marginalization of social groups, extreme poverty and disasters caused by natural phenomena, these lead to changes in the life of the patient itself, disfiguring the effect or impact that these situations also have on the caregivers.

It is detected late in most cases. Similarly, the importance of the role of informal caregivers in the well-being and care of the dependent person is recognized. In view of this problem, the conceptualization of burden proposed by the research conducted in Bucaramanga is based on the authors' definition of burden as "the experience resulting from the interrelation between the context of care and the characteristics of the patient, the coping resources, and the physical and emotional states of the informal caregiver of a dependent person" Zapata M 2019 (50).

The most common psychological and physical consequences for informal caregivers are found as time goes by and the caregiver assumes a great physical and psychological burden, as he/she takes full responsibility for the life of the patient (medication, medical visits, care, hygiene, food, etc.), gradually loses his/her independence as the patient takes up more and more of his/her time and neglects him/herself.), he gradually loses his independence as the patient absorbs more and more of his time and neglects himself, does not take the necessary free time for leisure, abandons his hobbies, does not go out with his friends, etc., and ends up paralyzing, for many years, his life project. Bedoya J (51).

With the time spent as a caregiver of a dependent person, the life disposition of the patient improves considerably, while the caregiver's life disposition is affected to the same extent; in this order of ideas, the family caregiver is mainly in charge of supplying the needs that the patient cannot satisfy on his own.

They live the process with high levels of stress, a great perception of burden that, sometimes, proliferates to several areas of life with serious consequences for their health appearing sleep disturbances, depression, stress, joint pain, headaches, suicidal behaviors and ideation, aggressiveness, substance abuse, inattention, low self-esteem, desires to abandon work (and care), denial of emotions or displacement of affections. And, finally, a worse immune response to the influence of vaccines, a matter of major importance in the midst of a pandemic. Falcone L 2021 (52).

All the aforementioned harmonizes with the idea of demand on the part of the caregiver, introducing him/her in a field that may affect his/her integrity from another aspect such as self-care, a concept that is related to the actions that are executed and that promote health; that lead to physical, mental and spiritual wellbeing.

At this point it is key to mention the theorist Henderson V (24) who belongs to those models that begin with the theory of the needs and health of human life as a central core for nursing.

According to this model, this person is a whole being, with biological, psychological, sociocultural and spiritual components that interact with each other and tend to develop to their maximum potential. V. Henderson believes that the main function of nursing is to help a person, healthy or ill, to maintain or restore health (or assist them in their last moments) in order to meet their needs.

In other words, Henderson V's theory (24) tries to explain that a person has needs that must be met in order to enjoy good health, so he identifies 14 basic needs, i.e., those needs that must be met by the person himself. or if there is a physical or mental disability, etc. They must be attended to by a guardian, who in this case will be in contact with the patient, not only to help him/her recover or maintain his/her health but also to ensure his/her comfort.

Henderson V (24) also tells us about the four elements of his theoretical model:

Health: defined by her as the capacity of a person to satisfy his or her needs in a totally independent manner, thus enjoying the highest quality of life.

Environment: all external conditions that can positively or negatively affect human health.

Human: considers the human being as a whole, a psychosocial being who must enjoy physical, mental and social health in order to have a quality life.

Nursing: This is temporary assistance for someone who lacks the ability, strength or knowledge to meet any of the 14 basic needs until the person is able to meet them on his or her own. Nursing care will aim to restore this independence from a point of view related to the research project, the nursing staff would become covered by a caregiver, either this formal and informal which may be a close relative, this subject would go on to fulfill the functions of caregiver towards an older adult, which requires support to meet their 14 physiological needs if required to obtain the best possible quality for the older adult or to assist the healthy or sick individual in carrying out activities that contribute to their health and well-being, recovery or to achieve a dignified death. Pastuña R 2020 (53).

The nursing professional has the ability to diagnose the individualized needs of the patient. It reaffirms the 14 basic needs of the human being. It contemplates 3 levels of intervention as: substitute, aid or companion.

In addition, the issue of caregiver resilience and caregiver overload focuses on the fact that the caregiver needs time to enjoy good health, knowing how to take good control of their needs as described by Virginia Henderson, so it is important to avoid caregiver overload at all costs, as it affects the health of both the caregiver and the older adult under their care and in a broader concept also affects their family, social and work environment.

Considering the above, the theory of Henderson V (24) has too much influence on the research work since it will mainly take into account activities such as:

- Movements and postures
- Drinking and eating properly
- Maintaining body hygiene
- Recreational activities

The Zarit scale is an instrument where results are obtained on the level of burden or fatigue of caregivers of people with dementia or dependence, as described by Zamora W 2021(54), it is a self-administered test where dimensions such as self-care capacity, quality of life, social support network and others are assessed.

This test consists of 22 items, in which the frequency is evaluated with values between 1 and 5, where 1 is never, 2 is rarely, 3 is sometimes, 4 is quite often and 5 is almost always. When these values are added together, the score ranges between 22 and 110 points. According to the results, the level of caregiver overload is classified as follows: absence of overload, when the score is less than or equal to 46 points, light overload from 47 to 55, and intense overload when the score is equal to or greater than 56.

7. LEGAL FRAMEWORK

- Political Constitution of Colombia. It is the fundamental law that governs our country. It guarantees the rights and freedoms of the people. It regulates the organization and exercise of the powers of the State 2022 (55).
- Republic of Colombia. Ministry of Social Protection. Law number 100 of 1993. The purpose of this comprehensive plan is to guarantee the inalienable rights of the individual and the community to obtain a quality of life in accordance with human dignity, through the protection of the contingencies that affect it (56).
- The Congress of Colombia. Law 33 of 2009. Defines the family caregiver as "the family caregiver shall be the person who, being the spouse, partner or permanent companion of the dependent person or having a relationship up to the fifth degree of consanguinity, third degree of affinity or first civil relationship with the same, demonstrates that he/she provides assistance" (57).
- The Congress of Colombia. Law 266 of 1996. Its purpose is to provide comprehensive health care to the individual, the family, the community and its environment; to help develop individual and collective potentials to the maximum, to maintain healthy living practices that will safeguard an optimal state of health at all stages of life (58).
- The Congress of Colombia. Law 1090 of 2006, article 2 numeral 9 referred to the research with humans and the respect for the dignity and welfare of the people who participate with full knowledge of the research. Likewise, the provisions of Article 50, which states that research conducted by psychology professionals must be based on the ethical principles of respect and dignity, and safeguard the welfare and rights of the participants (59), were also assumed.

- The Congress of Colombia. Law 1751 of 2015. through which the fundamental right to health is regulated provides in Article 5 that the State is responsible for respecting, protecting and guaranteeing the effective enjoyment of this right, as one of the essential elements of the Social State of Law, and in Article 10 states as duties of individuals to "promote their self-care, that of their family and their community" and to "act in solidarity in situations that endanger the life and health of people" (60).
- The Colombian Congress. Law 9 of 1979, highlights in its Title VII that it corresponds to the State as regulator in health matters, to issue the necessary provisions to ensure an adequate situation of hygiene and safety in all activities and in its article 598 establishes that, "every person must ensure the improvement, conservation and recovery of his personal health and the health of the members of his household, avoiding harmful actions and omissions and complying with the technical instructions and mandatory standards issued by the competent authorities" (61).
- Congress of Colombia. Ministry of health and social protection resolution number 005928 of 2016, by which the requirements for the recognition and payment of the caregiver service ordered by tutela ruling to the reimbursing entities are established, as an exceptional service financed from the resources of the General System of Social Security in Health the minister of health and social protection (62).
- Congress of the Republic of Colombia. Law 911, in Chapter I, Article 4, sets out the principles of nursing practice, namely: integrality, individuality, dialogicity, quality, continuity and states that the care process is directed at the person, family and community, which clearly shows that nursing has a role in community care (63).

8. METHODOLOGICAL DESIGN

8.1 Type of study.

For the development of this work, a cross-sectional descriptive analytical quantitative study was used. It seeks to know the overload of the main caregiver of patients with chronic diseases. For this purpose, information will be collected in the months of May and August 2023, in the aforementioned institution.

8.2 Population.

The population consisted of 120 caregivers of patients belonging to the complementary health care provider in Montería Córdoba 20232.

8.3 Inclusion Criteria .

- Informal caregiver of chronically ill patients.
- Person of legal age (18 years old)
- Caregivers providing unpaid care
- Caregivers who have more than three months caring for chronically ill patients.

8.4 Exclusion criteria .

- Caregiver with cognitive-behavioral problems
- Person who does not wish to participate in the study.

8.5 Instruments for data collection.

Two instruments were used in the present investigation: a sociodemographic survey and the Zarit burden scale test survey. Zamora W 2021(54).

8.5.1 Sociodemographic Characteristics Survey (Annex 1).

The sociodemographic survey was prepared by the research group and consists of eight items or questions with information on sex, origin, schooling, marital status, occupation, stratum, relationship with the caregiver and the number of hours dedicated to caregiving.

8.5.2 Zarit Load Test Scale (Annex 2).

The Zarit Caregiver Burden Test instrument. The Spanish version of Montorio et al. was used. It consists of 22 items that measure the burden perceived by the caregiver through a 4-point Likert scale, ranging from 0 (never), 1 (Rarely), 2 (Sometimes), 3 (Quite often), 4 (Almost always). Where the respondent must indicate the question with which he/she feels identified according to the above-mentioned statements. Adding the 22 questions, a single index of burden is obtained with a score range from 0 to 88 points.

Where a score of less than 47 points is obtained, there is no overload, scores of 47 to 55 points indicate mild overload and scores of more than 55 points indicate intense overload; this identifies that if the informal caregiver has a score of more than 47 points there is an urgent need to modify the way of caring for the family member and this caregiver requires help as soon as possible, in addition if scores of more than 55 points are obtained there is a high risk of diseases such as depression and anxiety.

The instrument was evaluated for its internal consistency, which obtained a Cronbach's alpha of greater than or equal to 0.9, its degree of validity and reliability 0.81 to 0.91 interval with 65% confidence.

8.6 Collection and statistical analysis:

Authorization was requested from the management of the primary health care provider where the information was to be collected using the aforementioned instruments; once this was obtained, the objectives of the study were explained to each potential participant in the present study and once they understood them, they proceeded to sign the informed consent form. Once the consent form was filled out, the two instruments that comprise the present study were filled out. The information was collected by the research group and its research teacher. Once the instruments were applied to the study sample, a database was created in Excel 2013, where the data obtained were included. For the analysis of the information, a statistical package SPSS version 22 was used, under IBM license, which allowed the analysis of descriptive statistics in frequencies and percentages.

9. VARIABLES

Table 1. Operationalization of the variables.

VARIABLE (DEFINITION)	DIMENSIONS	I1NDICATOR	ITEM	VARIABLE TYPE
SOCIODEMOGRAPHIC FACTORS OF THE CAREGIVER: It emphasizes the diversity of aspects that allow the person to interact with other people, for which the existence of others with self-awareness, language and the intention to communicate is essential. It is an essential component for life and human development as it is impossible	CAREGIVER SOCIAL FACTORS	STRATUM	Stratum 1	QUANTITATIVE
			Stratum 2	
			Stratum 3	
			Strata 4	
		OCCUPATION	Home	QUALITATIVE
			Employee	
			Self-employment	
			Student	
			Others	
		SCHOLARSHIP	Primary Incomplete	QUALITATIVE ORDINAL
			Completed elementary school	
			Incomplete	

to be human alone.			baccalaureate Completed baccalaureate Technician Complete University incomplete university	
	CAREGIVER DEMOGRAPHIC FACTORS	SEX	Female Male	QUALITATIVE DICHOTOMOUS
		CIVIL STATUS	Single Married Widower Free union	QUALITATIVE
CARE CONDITIONS: These refer to the material context in which the care	CHARACTERIZATION OF CARE CONDITIONS.	NUMBER OF HOURS YOU ARE IN CARE IN CARE	FROM 1 TO 6 HOURS FROM 6 TO 12	DISCRETE QUANTITATIVE

of the patient takes place.			HOURS	
			12 TO 18 HOURS	
			18 TO 24 HOURS	
		RELATIONSHIP WITH THE CAREGIVER:	SPOUSE (A)	QUALITATIVE
			MOTHER	
			FATHER	
			SON	
			GRANDFATHER	
			FRIEND (A)	
OVERLOAD (Zarit) The emotional, physical, social and economic suffering that occurs as a result of caring for a friend or family member	DEGREES OF OVERLOAD State resulting from the action of caring for a dependent person.	NO OVERLOAD	(≤46)	QUANTITATIVE
		LIGHT OVERLOAD	(47-55)	QUANTITATIVE
		HEAVY OVERLOAD	(≥56)	QUANTITATIVE

with a chronic illness or disability.				

10. ETHICAL CONSIDERATIONS

The present study established its ethical guidelines according to resolution 008430 of October 4, 1993. In accordance with this resolution, since it is a study involving human beings, respect for their dignity and the protection of their rights and well-being prevailed (64). In addition, the Helsinki declaration will be taken into account (65). The execution of this project will begin once the research committee of the nursing faculty of the Universidad del Sinú Elías Bechara Zainúm approves it.

These are framed within the consideration and respect for individuals, the consent to participate in the study, the avoidance of putting key informants at risk, the guarantee of data protection, and the responsibility and transparency of the research team.

On the other hand, we considered the ethical requirements proposed by Emanuel E (66) for research on human subjects:

Value: This research contributes to the empowerment of the nursing profession, as it will allow the identification of the imaginary meanings of the profession and the areas susceptible to intervention, it can also be a methodological reference for the fulfillment of the global leadership strategies of the profession.

Scientific validity: The present study is original, requiring minimal exposure of the participants. It has a valid methodological design and data analysis process.

Favorable risk-benefit ratio: The physical and emotional integrity of the key informants was respected; data protection, privacy and confidentiality of the information obtained from the interviews with the participants was guaranteed. For this purpose, proper names were not used; instead, a numbering system was designed for the interviews, categories and hypotheses obtained.

Independent evaluation: The study presented social accountability, the independent evaluation was conducted by the evaluation committee of the Nursing faculty of the Universidad del Sinú Elías Bechara Zainúm and the primary health care provider.

Informed consent: An informed consent form was prepared that provided information about the objectives of the study, the possible risks to which they were exposed and the benefits of the research, with the necessary elements to make a voluntary decision without coercion to participate. It was also explained that the study was conducted for academic purposes only.

The authors declare that they have no conflicts of interest with respect to the preparation, execution, authorship and subsequent publication of this project.

11. RESULTS

11.1 Socio-demographic characteristics

There were 120 informal caregivers, of which the predominant sex was female with 77% (92) followed by male with 23% (28), as for the origin the urban area with 69% (83) followed by rural with 31% (37), their schooling was predominantly high school with 48.2% (58) followed by technical or more with 32.5% (39) and lastly primary with 19.1% (23).1 (23), marital status predominated single with 36.6% (44), followed by married with 31.8% (37) as well as free union with 26.6% (32) and lastly separated/widowed and others 5.7% (7), in terms of occupation, housewife predominated with 42.5% (51) followed by independent worker with 27.5% (33) and also employee with 22.5% (27) and lastly, the last one with 27.5% (27).5% (27) and lastly student with 7.5% (9), level 1 predominates with 80% (96), followed by level 2 with 19.1% (23) and lastly level 3 with 0.8% (1), with regard to the relationship between the informal caregiver and the patient, it was observed that the relationship between the child predominates with 58.3% (70), followed by wife with 15% (18) and mother or father with 11.6% (14) and grandfather or grandmother with 11.6% (14) and grandfather or grandmother with 12.6% (14).6% (14) and grandfather or grandmother with 8.3% (10), as for the number of hours that the informal caregiver dedicates to the care of his/her relative, the number of hours from 6 to 12 hours predominated with 52.5% (63), followed by 12 to 18 hours with 25.8% (31) as well as from 1 to 6 hours with 13.3% (16) and finally the number of hours from 18 to 24 hours with 8.3% (10). (Table 1)

11.2. Degree of overload at the global level

The overburden of the informal caregiver of the population, at a global level according to the Zarit scale indicates that 66% (79) of the caregivers present no overburden, followed by 19% (23) with light overburden and 15% (18) with intense overburden; based on these results Zarit identifies that the population with light overburden needs to urgently modify their way of caring for the elderly person and requires help as soon as possible; likewise for the population with intense overburden they present a high risk of becoming ill with depression or anxiety (Table 2).

11.3 Functional dependence related to the number of hours dedicated to the care of the chronically ill patient.

The functional dependence of the chronic patient was calculated by the number of hours dedicated to care; it was observed that the greatest number of hours dedicated are from 6 to 18 hours daily to the care of the chronic patient, with this it is determined that the functional dependence of the patient is 78% (94), followed by 1 to 6 hours with functional dependence of 13% (16), and from 18 to 24 hours a functional dependence of 8% was observed (10). (Table 1).

11.4 Sex and overload relationship

In relation to overload with sex, it was observed that the female sex presented light and intense overload 27.5% (33) compared to the male sex with light and intense overload 6.6% (8). (Table 3)

11.5 Relationship of origin (urban/rural) and overburdening

In relation to overload with origin (urban/rural), it was observed that the origin that presented the greatest light and intense overload was the urban zone, 20.8% (25), compared to the rural zone with 13.3% (16). (Table 4)

11.6 Relationship of schooling with overload

In relation to overload with schooling, it was observed that the high school level presented the greatest light and intense overload 16.6% (20), followed by technical or more 9.1% (11). And incomplete elementary school 8.3% (10). (Table 5).

11.7 Relationship of marital status and overburdening

The relationship between overload and marital status was observed as follows: single, with a greater light and intense overload 11.6% (14), followed by free union 8.3% (10). (Table 6)

11.8 Relationship of occupancy and overload.

The relationship between overload and occupation showed that housewife presented a greater light and intense overload 19.1% (23), followed by independent worker 8.3% (10). And employee 5% (6). Table (7)

11.9 Stratum and overburden relationship

In relation to the overload with the stratum, it was observed that stratum 1 presents greater light and intense overload 27.5% (33), and level 2 with 5.8% (7). Table (8)

11.2.1 Relationship with the cared-for person and overload

In relation to overload with the caregiver, it was observed that the child presented greater light and intense overload 20.8% (25), and the spouse 5.8% (7). Table (9)

11.2.2. Relationship between number of hours dedicated to care and Overload

The relationship between overload and the number of hours dedicated to caregiving showed that 6-12 hours presented a greater light and intense overload 18.3% (22), and 12-18 hours 14.1% (17). (Table 10)

12. DISCUSSION

Informal caregiver overload in patients with chronic diseases is a phenomenon that has gained increasing attention in the field of health and wellness. Chronic diseases, characterized by their long duration and need for ongoing care, impact not only the lives of those who suffer from them, but also their informal caregivers. As the aging of the population and the prevalence of chronic diseases increase, it is crucial to understand the physical, emotional and social challenges faced by these caregivers (8), in this context the present research found globally that the overburden presented by informal caregivers is absence of overburden with 66%, followed by light overload 19% and finally 15% with overload, similar to what was found by Flores R 2020 (67), where it shows that at a global level in his study 99% of the population studied presented absence of overload and 1% with light overload. Contrary to what was found in the study of Rivas G 2022 (68), where 100% of the population studied presented light overload; likewise Amador C 2020 (69) reports that globally 74% of the population studied presented light overload.

Likewise, in the Zarit scale qualification for those patients who present slight overload with scores higher than 47 points need to urgently modify the way of caring for the older adult and require help. In addition, those patients who presented intense overload are at high risk of presenting depressive illnesses and anxiety (54).

Regarding the functional dependence of the chronic patient, a relationship was established through the number of hours that the informal caregiver dedicates to their integral care, observing that the patients with the greatest functional dependence are those who require care between 6 to 18 hours, establishing a functional dependence of 79%, followed by a functional dependence of 13% requiring from 1 to 6 hours of care, likewise 8% of functional dependence requires care from 18 to 24 hours of care; different from what was found in the study of Vega D where he reports that the functional dependence of patients with chronic diseases is 52.6% (70) Similar to Vega M's study where he found that 45.7% of his study population presented moderate functional dependence (71).

Although the aging of human populations is a universal phenomenon, demographic changes are occurring at a faster rate than in other countries due to the extraordinary decrease in fertility and the increase in life expectancy. These transformations are accompanied by the existence of people in need of care as a result of the dependency generated by the presence of a disabling disease, such as chronic diseases (12,28,35).

In this context, the informal caregiver is mainly the one who helps to meet the needs that his or her family member cannot meet on his or her own. He/she lives the process with high levels of stress, a great perception of burden that sometimes spreads to various areas of life with serious consequences for his/her health (24,46).

Regarding the sociodemographic characteristics of the surveyed population, it was observed that the predominant gender is female with 76.6%, a case similar to the findings of Zepeda P (72), where 74.4% are female, as well as in the research of Flores R (63), where 68.8% are female.

According to the schooling of those surveyed, 40.8% of the respondents had a high school level (baccalaureate), which is different from the study by Carrion D (73) where 56% of the population has higher education, another different study was the research by Tomala J where primary schooling predominated with 83% (74), a similar study was that of Guaman P where 25.9% (75) of the respondents had a high school level.

Regarding the marital status of the respondents, the single population predominated 36.6%, a similar study was that of Villalobos G, Pichardo M with 33.3% (76) different from the study by Rivas G, Tapahuasco K with 48.3% (64), Another different study was that of Agudelo M, Ayala M, Moreno M, Salón C, with 50%, (77).

Regarding the occupation of the respondents, the home was predominant with 42.5%, different from the study by Hernández A where 50% of the population is pensioned (78), different from the study by Flores R with 45.16% (63), another different study was that of Navarrete A, where students predominated with 25% (79).

According to the relationship with the cared-for person, the predominant relationship was Son with 58%, in contrast to the study by Hernández A, where the predominant relationship was Spouse with 50% (74), and another study by Guaman P, where the most relevant relationship was Other with 32.9% (80).

According to the number of hours dedicated to caring for the patient, it was from 6 to 12 hours with 52.5%, similar to the study of Romero E with 52.7% (81), different to the study found by Tomala J, less than 8 hours with 45% (82), another different study was that of Zepeda A, where 24 hours predominated with 72.97% (83).

Finally, one of the strengths evidenced in this study is to be a pioneer in the department of Córdoba in measuring the level of functional dependence of chronic patients with their caregivers, in addition to performing the statistical association between sociodemographic characteristics and levels of overload according to the Zarit test.

13. LIMITATIONS

The entity where the information was collected or the instrument was applied did not allow the researcher to have a closer approach with the caregivers, because they were accompanying their relatives to a medical appointment.

14. CONCLUSIONS

The overload of the informal caregiver in the primary health care provider, at a global level, presented an absence of overload, due to the complementary intra and/or extra institutional activities that the primary health care provider performs in the community. It should be noted that a small percentage of the population described in the results presented a slight overload that merits urgent modification of their way of caring and requires help; likewise, another small percentage presented an intense overload, who are at high risk of suffering from illnesses such as depression or anxiety.

The functional dependence of the chronic patient on his or her caregiver was established by the number of hours spent by the informal caregiver in his or her care, with a functional dependence ratio of 79%.

The results made it possible to meet the study objectives and identify a positive correlation between caregiving competencies and informal caregiver overload, which can be interpreted as "the higher the caregiving competencies, the lower the level of overload". These findings show that informal caregivers and primary health care providers have various competencies and skills to optimally exercise their roles as caregivers and health care providers and therefore have the ability to cope with situations of overload.

Therefore, the results of this study provide knowledge to generate nursing educational strategies to increase caregiving competencies and thereby decrease caregiver overload and the risk of developing diseases such as depression or anxiety and prevent complications in the people under their care.

15. RECOMMENDATIONS

For practice: Create self-help groups made up of informal caregivers to share experiences, thoughts and feelings, to overcome fears, resolve doubts and find and provide support.

For nursing: Promote and encourage the training of caregivers in the care that the patient should receive according to his/her pathology and make family members aware of the quality of care that the patient should receive.

Create a plan of home visits for caregivers of dependent older adults in order to follow up on the caregiver's health condition.

Health institution: Organize an easily accessible care route for the caregiver that is geared towards the delivery of medicines or necessary supplies required by the dependent older adult.

Distribute caregiving responsibilities among family members in order to decrease or prevent the presence of overburden.

To promote as much as possible the independence and autonomy of the dependent elderly.

For research: In the next studies, subjective and objective informal caregiver overload could be measured, thereby obtaining a broader analysis of the phenomenon under study.

16. BIBLIOGRAPHY .

1. World health organization 2021; aging and health. (Accessed March 23, 2023). Available at: https://www.who.int/es/news-room/fact-sheets/detail/ageing-and-health

2. Pardo Y, Chaparro L, Carreño S. Business plan for nursing interventions: "caring for caregivers" program. Cuidarte Rev. 2022; (Accessed March 23, 2023). Available at: http://dx.doi.org/10.15649/cuidarte.1994

3. Guato P, Mendoza S. Self-care of the informal caregiver of the elderly in some Latin American countries: descriptive review. Art. 2022. (Accessed March 23, 2023). Disponible en: http://www.scielo.edu.uy/pdf/ech/v11n2/2393-6606-ech-11-02-e2917.pdf

4. Fernández B, Herrera S. Health effects of dependent older people caregiving by family members. Rev 2020. (Accessed March 23, 2023). Disponible en: https://www.scielo.cl/pdf/rmc/v148n1/0717-6163-rmc-148-01-0030.pdf

5. Cárdenas D. Overload syndrome and quality of life of the caregiver of patients with disabilities in the first level of care. MS thesis. Universidad Técnica de Ambato/Facultad de Ciencias de la Salud/Centro de Posgrados 2022. (Accessed March 24, 2023). Available at: https://repositorio.uta.edu.ec/bitstream/123456789/34900/1/%c3%a1rdenas_paredes_diana_ver%c3%b3nica.pdf

6. Abdellatif O, Abderrahmane A, Fatiha C. Assessment of the burden placed on caregivers of patients with dementia using the ZARIT-MOR scale in Morocco 2022. (Accessed March 26, 2023). Available at: https://ibdigital.uib.es/greenstone/sites/localsite/collect/medicinaBalear/index/assoc/AJHS_Med/icina_Ba/lear_202/3v38n2p0/31.dir/AJHS_Medicina_Balear_2023v38n2p031.pdf
7. Martinez S. Informal caregiver overload syndrome 2020. (Accessed March 26, 2023). Available at: https://scielo.isciii.es/pdf/ene/v14n1/1988-348X-ene-14-1-e14118.pdf

8. Murillo D, Fernandez E, Velasco E. Chronic patient care and case management in nursing 2019. (Accessed March 29, 2023). Available at: https://www.editdiazdesantos.com/wwwdat/pdf/9788490522196.pdf

9. Celeiro T, Galizzi. M. Quality of life in institutionalized and non-institutionalized older adults aged 70-85 years in the city of Nogoyá. 2019. (Accessed March 29, 2023). Available at: https://repositorio.uca.edu.ar/bitstream/123456789/9721/1/calidad-vida-adultos-mayores-70.pdf

10. Ulloa O, Martínez L, Hernández K, Fernández L. Immobility syndrome in older adults of the Bernardo Posse Polyclinic of the San Miguel del Padrón municipality 2019. (Accessed March 29, 2023). Disponible en: http://scielo.sld.cu/pdf/gme/v21n3/1608-8921-gme-21-03-30.pdf

11.Menéndez T, Génesis L, Caicedo L. "Stress as a main factor of the caregiver syndrome in representatives of people with disabilities of the FADINNAF foundation 2019. Rev (Accessed March 29, 2023). Available at: https://www.eumed.net/rev/caribe/2019/01/estres-sindrome-cuidador.html

12.Aguinaga S, Perez D. Grief and complicated bereavement: A review of the scientific literature over time. Rev 2022. (Accessed March 29, 2023). Available at: file:///C:/Users/ORHEX/AppData/Local/Microsoft/Windows/INetCache/IE/R39OOFW4/210-Text%20of%20art%20C3%ADculo-896-2-10-20220103[1].pdf.

13.Gonzalez C. Personality dimensions and their relationship to psychological well-being in caregivers of persons with disabilities 2022. (Accessed June 12, 2023). Available at: https://repositorio.uta.edu.ec/bitstream/123456789/34782/1/Gonzalez%20Catota%20Carla%20Mariela%20-%20Repositorio.pdf

14.Serra M. Chronic noncommunicable diseases and the COVID-19 pandemic. Art 2020. (Accessed June 12, 2023). Available at: https://www.medigraphic.com/pdfs/finlay/fi-2020/fi202c.pdf

15.Noa Y, Coll J, Echemendia A. Atividade física no adulto mais velho com doenças crónicas não transmissíveis. Rev Podium 2021 . Art. (Accessed June 19, 2023). Disponible en: http://scielo.sld.cu/pdf/rpp/v16n1/1996-2452-rpp-16-01-308.pdf

16.Arias C, Muñoz M. Quality of life and overload in caregivers of schoolchildren with intellectual disabilities 2019. (Accessed June 19, 2023). Available at: http://www.scielo.org.ar/pdf/interd/v36n1/v36n1a17.pdf

17.Hernández J, Jiménez A, Pérez I. Transcendence of communication in the quality of life of older adults in social distancing by COVID-19. Journal 2022. (Accessed June 19, 2023). Available at: https://www.revistadecomunicacionysalud.es/index.php/rcys/article/view/288/356

18.De La Serna J, Moreno A, Cremaschi F. Parkinson's disease: late stages 2020. Book (Accessed June 28, 2023). Available at: https://books.google.es/books?hl=en&lr=&id=w0YQEAAAAQBAJ&oi=fnd&pg=PT3&dq=+Parkinson's+disease:+%C3%BAlast+stages&ots=vI6AYvXYgk&sig=oHBbV_DRIhhzXMMWVVGc8GjbCFrY#v=onepage&q=Disease%20of%20parkinson%3A%20%C3%BAlast%20stages&f=false.

19.Menéndez T, Génesis L, Caicedo L. "Stress as a main factor of the caregiver syndrome in representatives of people with disabilities of the FADINNAF foundation 2019. Rev (Accessed June 30, 2023). Available at: https://www.eumed.net/rev/caribe/2019/01/estres-sindrome-cuidador.html

20.Cárdenas C. Primary Health Care. Outreach to families of breast cancer patients. Revista 2021. (Accessed August 2, 2023). Available at: https://psicologiacientifica.com/atencion-primaria-familias-pacientes-con-cancer/

21.Rabelo A. Factors associated with the psychological well-being of caregivers of people with disabilities. Research article (Psychology), Faculty of Human, Social and Educational Sciences, Pereira, 2022. (Accessed August 03, 2023). Available at: https://repositorio.ucp.edu.co/bitstream/10785/12061/1/DDMPSI404.pdf

22.Sas c. what were the leading causes of death Colombia 2022? 2023 (Accessed August 03, 2023). Available at: https://consultorsalud.com/principales-causas-muerte-colombia-2022/

23.Garcia Y, Arias E, Salazar A. Predictors of quality of life in caregivers of patients with chronic disease. Revista 2022. (Accessed August 03, 2023). Available at: https://dialnet.unirioja.es/servlet/articulo?codigo=8801244

24.Cruz L. Caregiver overload and perceived social support in caregivers of older adults 2022. (Accessed August 03, 2023). Available at: https://repositorio.ucv.edu.pe/bitstream/handle/20.500.12692/95004/Cruz_BLJ-SD.pdf?sequence=4&isAllowed=y

25.Henderson V. Definition of nursing and the 14 components of nursing care 2008.(Accessed August 03, 2023). Available at: https://slsucoam.blogspot.com/2008/09/definition-of-nursing-and-14-components.html?m=1

26.Doicela R, Jara P. The search for nursing autonomy from virginia Henderson's point of view. 2020. (Accessed August 08, 2023). Available at: https://revistas.uta.edu.ec/erevista/index.php/enfi/article/view/975/906

27.Elso R, Solis L. The process of nursing care in out-of-hospital emergencies. (Accessed August 08, 2023). Disponible en: https://www.codem.es/Adjuntos/CODEM/Documentos/Informaciones/Publico/9e8140e2-cec7-4df7-8af9-8843320f05ea/8c06b7e5-ca29-40c6-ab63-f84959a87362/c618e862-974d-4faf-8093-66eae984e3da/TRABAJO_CONGRESO_GRAFICA_AJUSTADA.pdf

28.Arias E, Carreño S, Chaparro O. Uncertainty in the face of chronic disease. Integrative review. 2019. (Accessed August 20, 2023). Available at: https://bibliotecadigital.udea.edu.co/bitstream/10495/21358/1/AriasEdier_2019_IncertidumbreEnfermedadCr%c3%b3nica.pdf

29.Sierra L, Montoya R, Garcia M, Lopez M, Montalvo A. Family caregiver experience with palliative and end-of-life care. 2019. (Accessed August 12, 2023). Available at:

https://scielo.isciii.es/scielo.php?pid=S1132-12962019000100011&script=sci_arttext

30.Guerrero D, Carreño S, Chaparro L. Family caregiver overload in Colombia: an exploratory systematic review. Rev. 2023. (Accessed August 12, 2023). Available at: https://revistacolombianadeenfermeria.unbosque.edu.co/index.php/RCE/article/view/3754/3554

31.Aguado E. Profile of the caregiver of the patient with Chronic Kidney Disease: a review of the literature. Enferm Nefrol 2019. (Accessed August 12, 2023). Available at: https://scielo.isciii.es/pdf/enefro/v22n4/2255-3517-enefro-22-04-352.pdf

32.Esquivel N, Carreño S, Chaparro Lorena. Role of the novice family caregiver of dependent adults: scoping review. Revista 2021. (Accessed August 12, 2023). Available at: http://www.scielo.org.co/pdf/cuid/v12n2/2346-3414-cuid-12-2-e1368.pdf

33.Baracaldo H, Naranjo A, Medina V. Functional dependency level of institutionalized elderly people in welfare centers in Floridablanca (Santander, Colombia). 2019 (Accessed May 15, 2023). Disponible en: https://scielo.isciii.es/scielo.php?script=sci_arttext&pid=s1134-928x2019000400163#:~:text=seg%c3%ban%20la%20organizaci%c3%b3n%20mundial%20de,de%20los%20m%c3%a1rgenes%20normales%e2%80%9d2.

34. Salinas A, Manrique B, Montañez C. Effect of caregiver overload on the association between disability and quality of life in older adults. 2022. (Accessed May 16, 2023). Available at: https://www.medigraphic.com/pdfs/salpubmex/sal-2022/sal225h.pdf

35. Zuluaga M, Galeano M, Giraldo C, Vélez V, Sánchez S, et al. Meanings of care constructed by caregivers of the elderly. Rev. 2021. (Accessed May 16, 2023). Available at: https://revistas.ufps.edu.co/index.php/cienciaycuidado/article/view/2741/2954

36. Rivera M, Guerrero V. Quality of life in caregivers of patients with spinal cord injury. A documentary review. 2021. (Accessed May 16, 2023). Available at: http://repositorio.uan.edu.co/bitstream/123456789/2158/1/2020MarianaAlexandraRiveraFranco.pdf

37. Martínez L, Llantá M. Caregiver burden in primary informal caregivers of patients with head and neck cancer. Rev 2019. (Accessed May 18, 2023). Available at: http://scielo.sld.cu/pdf/rhcm/v18n1/1729-519X-rhcm-18-01-126.pdf

38. Mora B. Burden, depression and facilitation in Colombian informal caregivers of patients with schizophrenia and patients with dementia. 2020. (Accessed May 16, 2023). Available at: https://www.researchgate.net/profile/Belvy-Mora-Castaneda/publication/357057458_carga_depresion_y_familismo_en

_cuidadores_informales_colombianos_de_pacientes_con_esquizofrenia_y_pacientes_con_demencia_1/links/61ba0d08fd2cbd7200a17c08/carga-depresion-y-familismo-en-cuidadores-informalescolombianos-de-pacientes-con-esquizofrenia-y-pacientes-con-demencia-1.pdf

39. Soriano I, Castrejón R, Ávila L. León M, Toledano L, et al. Primary caregiver overload in patients with terminal cancer. 2022. (Accessed May 19, 2023). Available at: https://www.medigraphic.com/pdfs/atefam/af-2022/af222c.pdf

40. Navarro M, Medina P, Hernández R, Correa S, Peralta S, Rubí M. Degree of Overload and Characterization of Caregivers of Older Adults with Diabetes Mellitus type 2. 2019 (Accessed May 20, 2023). Available at: https://revistas.um.es/eglobal/article/view/361401/271401

41. Garcia A. Caring for dependent elderly people and caregiver stress. Degree thesis. University of cantabria. Faculty of nursing 2019. (Accessed May 30, 2023). Available at: https://repositorio.unican.es/xmlui/bitstream/handle/10902/16476/GarciaPooAna.pdf?sequence=1&isAllowed=y

42. Hurtado D, Losardo R, Bianchi R. Full and integral health: a broader concept of health. Art. 2021. (Accessed May 30, 2023). Available at: https://www.ama-med.org.ar/uploads_archivos/2147/Rev-1-2021_pag-18-25_Losardo.pdf

43. Secretaría Distrital de Salud - SDS Information on affiliation to the general social security health system. 2023 (Accessed May 30, 2023). Available at: https://bogota.gov.co/servicios/guia-de-tramites-y-servicios/informacion-sobre-afiliacion-al-sistema-general-de-seguridad-social-en-salud

44. Tinoco A. Defining cancer: a scientific controversy between the orthodox and the critical paradigm in oncology. Art 2019. (Accessed May 30, 2023). Available at: https://revistas.unbosque.edu.co/index.php/rcfc/article/view/2271/2210

45. Pastora G, Ruperti J, Schwerzmannb Adults with congenital heart disease during the COVID-19 pandemic: ? at-risk population. Art 2020. (Accessed August 2, 2023). Available at: https://www.ncbi.nlm.nih.gov/pmc/articles/PMC7386304/pdf/main.pdf

46. Canchos M. Factors related to stroke in patients attended by emergency at the Hospital Nacional arzobispo Loayza - 2018. Thesis Universidad Nacional Mayor de San Marcos 2019. (Accessed August 4, 2023). Available at: http://38.43.142.130/bitstream/handle/20.500.12672/10368/Canchos_cm.pdf?sequence=3&isAllowed=y

47. Urbina Y, Carrera G, Quintana O, Guama L. Activity and treatment of rheumatoid arthritis. Rev 2020. (Accessed August 6, 2023). Disponible en: http://scielo.sld.cu/pdf/rcur/v22n3/1817-5996-rcur-22-03-e856.pdf

48. World Health Organization. Global action plan for the prevention and control of noncommunicable diseases 2013-2020. (Accessed August 4, 2023). Available at: https://www.asivamosensalud.org/actualidad/enfermedades-cronicas-una-epidemia-segun-la-oms#:~:text=Pandemia%20medicalizada&text=Cardiovasculares%20(for%20example%2C%20the%20infarcts,population%%C3%B3n%20of%20all%20the%20world.

49. Lorca M, Candia C. Aging, motor disability and exclusion. Rev. 2021 (Accessed August 6, 2023). Available at: http://revistascientificas.filo.uba.ar/index.php/runa/article/view/8197/9201

50. Zapata M, Montoya V, Rodríguez L, Foronda L. Experiences and training of informal caregivers of patients in the municipality of Envigado. 2019. (Accessed August 6, 2023). Disponible en: https://repository.ces.edu.co/bitstream/handle/10946/4856/1010030559_2020.pd;jsessionid=ECB3F0B496A46AB0F78867B88449BD64?sequence=5

51.Bedoya J. Risk and protective factors affecting the psychological well-being of four family caregivers of functionally dependent older adults in the municipality of Carepa, Antioquia 2022. (Accessed August 6, 2023). Available at: https://bibliotecadigital.udea.edu.co/bitstream/10495/31018/1/BedoyaJhon_2022_CuidadorAdultoMayor.pdf

52.Falcone L. Relationship between personal characteristics and the level of self-care according to the degree of caregiver burden of chronically ill caregivers in a Provincial Institution of the City of Rosario 2021. (Accessed August 8, 2023). Available at: http://biblioteca.puntoedu.edu.ar/bitstream/handle/2133/24645/PTE2280-FalconeC-2021.pdf?sequence=3&isAllowed=y

53.Pastuña R, Jara P. Pastuña R/Enfermería Investiga, Investigación, Vinculación, Docencia y Gestión-Vol. 5 No 4 2020. The search for nursing autonomy from the viewpoint of Virginia Henderson. Rev. 2020. (Accessed August 10, 2023). Available at: https://revistas.uta.edu.ec/erevista/index.php/enfi/article/view/975/906

54.Zamora W, Figueroa DC. Indiscriminate use of the Zarit instrument in caregivers of non-geriatric, non-demented chronic patients. Art 2021. (Accessed August 11, 2023). Available at: https://revistas.unab.edu.co/index.php/medunab/article/view/4059/3451

55. Political Constitution of Colombia, July 20, 1991 (accessed July 28, 2023). Available at: http://www.secretariasenado.gov.co/constitucion-politica

56. Republic of Colombia. Ministry of Social Protection. Law number 100 of 1993 (accessed July 28, 2023). Available at: https://www.minsalud.gov.co/sites/rid/lists/bibliotecadigital/ride/de/dij/ley-100-de-1993.pdf

57. The Congress of Colombia. Law 33 of 2009 (accessed July 28, 2023). Available at: https://vlex.com.co/vid/proyecto-ley-senado-451467698

58. The Congress of Colombia. Law 266 of 1996 (accessed July 28, 2023). Available at: https://www.mineducacion.gov.co/1759/articles-105002_archivo_pdf.pdf

59. Congress of Colombia. Law 1090 of 2006 (accessed July 28, 2023). Available at: https://www.funcionpublica.gov.co/eva/gestornormativo/norma.php?i=66205

60. The Congress of Colombia. Law 1751 of 2015. (accessed July 28, 2023). Available at: https://www.minsalud.gov.co/normatividad_nuevo/ley%201751%20de%202015.pdf

61. The Congress of Colombia. Law 9 of 1979 (accessed July 28, 2023). Available at: https://www.minsalud.gov.co/normatividad_nuevo/ley%200009%20de%201979.pdf

62. The Minister of Health and Social Protection. Resolution 005928 of 2016(accessed July 28, 2023). Available at: https://www.minsalud.gov.co/sites/rid/Lists/BibliotecaDigital/RIDE/DE/DIJ/resolucion-5928-de-2016.pdf

63. Congress of the Republic of Colombia. Law 911 of 2004, code of ethics of the nursing profession. Available at http://www.secretariasenado.gov.co/senado/basedoc/ley_0911_2004.html

64. Republic of Colombia. Ministry of Social Protection. Resolution number 8430 of 1993. By which the scientific, technical and administrative norms for health research are established. (Accessed August 26, 2021). Available at: https://www.minsalud.gov.co/sites/rid/Lists/BibliotecaDigital/RIDE/DE/DIJ/RESOLUCION-8430-DE-1993.PDF

65. World Medical Association Declaration of Helsinki (2013), ethical principles for medical research involving human subjects section, paragraphs 17-23. Available at: https://www.wma.net/es/policies-post/declaracion-de-helsinki-de-la-amm-principios-eticos-para-las-investigaciones-medicas-en-seres-humanos/

66. Emanuel E. What makes clinical research ethical. Seven ethical requirements. (Accessed April 26, 2021). Available at: https://www.bioeticacs.org/iceb/seleccion_temas/investigacionEnsayosClinicos/Emanuel_Siete_Requisitos_Eticos.pdf

67. Flores R. Impact of primary caregiver overload syndrome of geriatric patients on family functionality in patients of UMF 244 Ferrocarriles. National Autonomous University of Mexico. 2020. (Accessed 24 August 2023). Disponible en: https://ru.dgb.unam.mx/bitstream/20.500.14330/TES01000806762/3/0806762.pdf

68. Rivas G, Tapahuasco K. Family caregiver overload of chronically ill patients attending the Raul Porras Barrenechea Health Center - Carabayllo. Universidad Cesar Vallejo. 2022. (Accessed August 24, 2023). Available in: Rivas MGDJ-Tapahuasco VKD - SD.pdf (ucv.edu.pe).

69. Amador C, Puello E, Valencia N. Psychoaffective characteristics and overload of informal care of terminal oncology patients Monteria, Colombia. Rev. Cubana de salud pública. 2020; 46 (1): 14 63. (Accessed August 24 2023). Available at: https://www.scielosp.org/pdf/rcsp/2020.v46n1/e1463/es

70. Vega D, Ruiz A, Vaillant T. Burden in primary informal caregivers in adults in chronic neurological diseases. Rev. Cubana Salud Publica

2019; 15 (2): e1510. (Accessed 7 September 2023). Available at: https://www.scielosp.org/pdf/rcsp/2019.v45n2/e1510/es

71. Vega M. Family Caregiver Overload and Degree of Functional Dependence of the Patient with Cerebral Vascular Disease, Hospital La Caleta, Chimbote, Universidad Cesar Vallejo Perú 2021. (Accessed September 7, 2023). Available at: https://repositorio.ucv.edu.pe/bitstream/handle/20.500.12692/73310/Vega_AMR-SD.pdf?sequence=1&isAllowed=y

72. Zepete P, Muños C. Overload in primary caregivers of older adults with severe dependency in primary health care. 2019; 30 (1): (Accessed August 30 2023). Available at: https://scielo.isciii.es/pdf/geroko/v30n1/1134-928X-geroko-30-01-00002.pdf

73. Carrion D. Level of overload of the primary caregiver of oncologic patients at the regional clinical surgical teaching hospital. National university of callao 2019. (Accessed August 30 2023). Available at: http://repositorio.unac.edu.pe/bitstream/handle/20.500.12952/5379/ROMERO%2c%20MIUEL%2c%20FALCON%20FCS%202DA%20ESPE%202019.pdf?sequence=1&isAllowed=y

74. Tomala J. Caregiver overload in family members of older adults with chronic noncommunicable diseases. comuna bambil collao, 2021. Peninsula de Santa Elena State University. Research work. (Accessed August 31, 2023). Available at:

https://repositorio.upse.edu.ec/bitstream/46000/7130/1/UPSE-TEN-2022-0029.pdf

75.Guaman P. "Evaluation of overload to the caregiver of disabled patients through Zarit and Gijon, health center n°1 Ibarra, 2018. Universidad técnica del norte. Degree work (Accessed August 31, 2023). Disponible en: http://repositorio.utn.edu.ec/bitstream/123456789/9342/2/06%20ENF%201042%20TRABAJO%20GRADO.pdf

76.Villalobos G, Pichardo M. Primary caregiver overload of children with onco-hematologic disease attending the association for the fight against childhood cancer in 2019. (Accessed August 31 2023). Available at: https://www.kerwa.ucr.ac.cr/bitstream/handle/10669/88029/FINAL%20TFG.pdf?sequence=1&isAllowed=y

77.Agudelo M, Ayala M, Moreno M, Salon C. Level of overload of the primary caregiver of a family member diagnosed with cancer. Degree work. Cooperative University of Colombia (Accessed August 31, 2023). Available at: https://repository.ucc.edu.co/server/api/core/bitstreams/6aa6527b-39ff-4b48-82b2-2da16e8c95d5/content

78.Hernández A. Program for stress management, reduction of perceived burden and use of active coping in informal primary caregivers of patients with suspected Alzheimer's dementia. Degree work 2015.

(Accessed August 31 2023). Available at: https://riudg.udg.mx/bitstream/20.500.12104/91198/1/MCUCS10169.pdf

79.Navarrete A, Taipe A. Primary caregiver overload of patients with physical disabilities 2023. Article (Accessed August 31, 2023). Available at: https://saludconciencia.com.ar/index.php/scc/article/view/14/11

80.Guamán P. Evaluation of overload to the caregiver of disabled patients through Zarit and Gijón, health center n°1 Ibarra, 2018. (Accessed August 31 2023). Disponible en:http://repositorio.utn.edu.ec/bitstream/123456789/9342/2/06%20ENF%201042%20TRABAJO%20GRADO.pdf

81.Romero E, Bonilla M, Travezaño F. Level of overload of the primary caregiver of oncology patients at the regional clinical-surgical teaching hospital "Daniel Alcides Carrión - Huancayo 2019. (Accessed August 31, 2023). Available at: http://repositorio.unac.edu.pe/bitstream/handle/20.500.12952/5379/ROMERO%2c%20MIGUEL%2c%20FALCON%20FCS%202DA%20ESPE%202019.pdf?sequence=1&isAllowed=y

82.Tomala J. Caregiver overload in family members of older adults with chronic noncommunicable diseases. 2021. (Accessed August 31, 2023). Available at:

https://repositorio.upse.edu.ec/bitstream/46000/7130/1/UPSE-TEN-2022-0029.pdf

83.Zepeda A. Overload in primary caregivers of older adults with severe dependency in primary health care. (Accessed August 31, 2023). Available at: https://scielo.isciii.es/pdf/geroko/v30n1/1134-928X-geroko-30-01-00002.pdf

Table 1. Sociodemographic characteristics

Variables	Feature	Frequency	Percentage
Sex	Female	92	77%
	Male	28	23%
Source	Rural	37	31%
	Urban	83	69%
Schooling	Primary Incomplete	10	8%
	Primary	13	11%
	Incomplete Baccalaureate	20	17%
	Completed Baccalaureate	38	32%
	Technical or more	39	33%
Marital Status	Married	37	31%
	Separated	5	4%
	Single	44	37%
	Free union	32	27%
	Widower	1	1%

	Another	1	1%
Occupation	Employee	27	23%
	Student	9	8%
	Home	51	43%
	Self-Employed	33	28%
Stratum	Level 1	96	80%
	Level 2	23	19%
	Level 3 or more	1	1%
Relationship with the caregiver	Grandma	10	8%
	Friend	8	7%
	Spouse	18	15%
	Son	70	58%
	Mother/father	14	12%
Number of hours dedicated to patient care	1 - 6 hours	16	13%
	6 - 12 hours	63	53%
	12 - 18 hours	31	26%
	18 - 24 hours	10	8%

Source: Survey of informal caregiver of chronic patient in a primary health care pres tator.

Table 2. Overall level of overload

Overload	Frequency	Percentage
Absence of overload	79	66%
Light overload	23	19%
Intense overload	18	15%

Source: Survey conducted with informal caregiver of chronic patient at a primary health care provider.

Table 3. Sex * Overload Relationship

		Overload			Total
		Absence of overload	Light overload	Intense overload	
Sex	Male	20	5	3	28
	Female	59	18	15	92
Total		79	23	18	120

Source: Survey conducted with informal caregiver of chronic patient at a primary health care provider.

Table 4. Source * Overload Relationship

		Overload			Total
		Absence of overload	Light overload	Intense overload	
Source	Rural	21	9	7	37
	Urban	58	14	11	83
Total		79	23	18	120

Source: Survey conducted with informal caregiver of chronic patient at a primary health care provider.

Table 5. Relationship between Schooling * Overload

		Overload			Total
		Absence	Slight	Intense	
Schooling	Primary	10	2	1	13
	Incomplete elementary school	3	4	3	10
	Completed baccalaureate	26	7	5	38
	Incomplete baccalaureate	12	3	5	20
	Technical or more	28	7	4	39
Total		79	23	18	120

Source: Survey conducted with informal caregiver of chronic patient at a primary health care provider.

Table 6. Relationship Marital Status * Overload

		Overload			Total
		Absence	Slight	Intense	
Marital Status	Single	30	7	7	44
	Married	22	9	6	37
	Separated	4	1	0	5
	Widower	0	1	0	1
	Free union	22	5	5	32
	Other	1	0	0	1
Total		79	23	18	120

Source: Survey of informal caregiver of chronic patient at a primary health care provider.

Table 7. Occupancy * Overload Ratio

		Overload			Total
		Absence	Slight	Intense	
Occupation	Home	28	12	11	51
	Employee	21	3	3	27

	Self-employed	23	6	4	33
	Student	7	2	0	9
Total		79	23	18	120

Source: Survey conducted with informal caregiver of chronic patient at a primary health care provider.

Table 8. Stratum * Overburden Relationship

		Overload			Total
		Absence	Slight	Intense	
Stratum	Level 1	63	18	15	96
	Level 2	16	4	3	23
	Level 3 or more	0	1	0	1
Total		79	23	18	120

Source: Survey conducted with informal caregiver of chronic patient at a primary health care provider.

Table 9. Relationship with the caregiver * Overburdening

		Overload			Total
		Absence	Slight	Intense	
Relationship with the caregiver	Spouse	11	4	3	18
	Grandma	7	3	0	10
	Mother/father	9	3	2	14
	Son	45	13	12	70
	Friend	7	0	1	8
Total		79	23	18	120

Source: Survey conducted with informal caregiver of chronic patient at a primary health care provider.

Table 10. Relationship Number of hours dedicated to care * Overload

		Overload			Total
		Absence	Slight	Intense	
Number of hours	1 - 6 hours	15	1	0	16
	6-12 hours	41	11	11	63

dedicated to care	12-18 hours	14	10	7	31
	18 -24 hours	9	1	0	10
Total		79	23	18	120

Source: Survey of informal caregivers of chronic patients in a primary health care provider.

17. ANNEXES

ANNEX 1. SOCIODEMOGRAPHIC SURVEY .

Sociodemographic survey of primary caregiver care conditions.

Sex	**Reply**
Male	
Female	
Source	**Reply**
Rural	
Urbana	
Schooling	**Reply**
Primary	
Primary Incomplete	
Completed baccalaureate	
Incomplete Baccalaureate	
Technician/Technologist	
University	
Postgraduate other	
CIVIL STATUS	**Reply**
Single	
Married	
Separated	
Widower	
free union	
Occupation	**Reply**
Home	
Employee	
Self-employed	
Student	
Stratum	
Level 1	
Level 2	
Level 3 or more	
Relationship with the caregiver	**Reply**
Spouse	
Grandma	
Mother/father	
Son	
Friend	

Number of hours dedicated to care	**Reply**
1 - 6 hours	
6 - 12 hours	
12 - 18 hours	
18 - 24 hours	

APPENDIX 2. TEST ON CAREGIVER BURDEN (ZARIT AND ZARIT)

Zarit Caregiver Overload Scale (Caregiver Burde Interview)

This instrument assesses the overload perceived by the caregiver by means of 22 items, which evaluate the caregiver-patient relationship, health status, psychological well-being, finances and social life. It has a degree of validity and reliability of 0.81 to 0.91 of interval with 65% confidence, the consistency presented an alpha of 0.87. The evaluation of each item is made by means of a lickert scale ranging from 0 to 4, according to the presence or intensity of an affirmative answer, where (0) never, (1) almost never, (2) sometimes, (3) quite often and (4) almost always. The exception is the last dimension, in which the respondent is asked if he/she feels overwhelmed as a caregiver and the answers are (0) no, (1) a little, (2) moderate, (3) a lot and (4) extremely.

To perform the interpretation of the results, the lickert-type responses range from 0 to 4, where the results are summed into a total score ranging from 0 to 88 points, this result classifies the caregiver into: "no overload" (=46), "light overload" (47-55) and "intense overload" (=56).

Each item is scored as follows: Score for each item (add them all together for the result).

Frequency	Score
Never	0
Almost never	1
Sometimes	2
Quite often	3

Almost always	4

Ite m	Question to ask	Score
1	Do you feel that your family member is asking for more help than he/she really needs?	
2	Do you feel that because of the time you spend with your family member you no longer have enough time for yourself?	
3	Do you feel tense when you have to care for your family member and attend to other responsibilities?	
4	Are you embarrassed by your family member's behavior?	
5	Do you feel angry when you are near your family member?	
6	Do you think the current situation negatively affects your relationship with friends and other family members?	
7	Do you fear for the future of your family member?	
8	Do you feel that your family member depends on you?	
9	Do you feel overwhelmed when you have to be with your family member?	
10	Do you feel that your health has suffered as a result of caring for your family member?	

11	Do you feel that you do not have the private life you would like because of your family member?	
12	Do you think your social life has been affected by having to care for your family member?	
13	Do you feel uncomfortable inviting friends to your home because of your family member?	
14	Do you think your family member expects you to take care of him or her, as if you were the only person he or she can count on?	
15	Do you feel that you do not have enough money to care for your family member in addition to your other expenses?	
16	Do you feel that you will be unable to care for your family member for much longer?	
17	Do you feel that you have lost control over your life since your family member's illness manifested itself?	
18	Would you like to be able to entrust the care of your family member to others?	
19	Do you feel unsure about what to do with your family member?	
20	Do you feel you should do more than you do for your family member?	
21	Do you think you could take better care of your family member than you do?	
22	In general: do you feel overburdened by having to take care of your family member?	

ANNEX 3. INFORMED CONSENT

INFORMED CONSENT

Yo,

____

____

Identified with identification document N°____________________________________De ____________________, I accept to participate **VOLUNTARILY**, in the research called **"OVERLOADING OF THE INFORMAL CAREGIVER IN PATIENTS WITH CHRONIC ILLNESSES, IN A PRIMARY HEALTH CARE PROVIDER. MONTERÍA - CÓRDOBA, 2023".**

To be held during the first half of this year.

The names of the persons and all information provided will be treated privately and with strict confidentiality, these are consolidated in a database as part of the investigative work and respecting the current regulations of the HABEAS DATA law. Only global information of the investigation will be disclosed in a report in which the names of the persons from whom information is obtained will be omitted. In case there are expenses during the development of the investigation, they will be covered by the investment budget.

For the record, I sign my handwriting, this _______ day of the month of ______________ of 2023.

FIRMA ____

ANNEX 4. BUDGET

INPUTS	**QUANTITY**	**VALUE**	**TOTAL**
PRINTER CARTRIDGES	2	29.000 34.000	63.000
TRANSPORTATION FOR ACCESSORY TRANSPORTATION TO AND FROM THE SITE	3	150.000 120.000 60.000	330.000
BOLIGRAFOS	3	1.500	4.500
REAMS OF LETTER SIZE PAPER	2	20.000	40.000
INTERNET	3	60.000 60.000 60.000	180.000
STATISTIC	1	300.000	300.000
TOTAL			**917.500**

ANNEX 5. TIMELINE.

Schedule of activities.

SCHEDULE OF ACTIVITIES											
Activity	**Months (February - December 2023)**										
	Feb	**Sea**	**Apr**	**May**	**Jun**	**Jul**	**Agos**	**Sep.**	**Oct**	**Nov**	**Dec**
Bibliographic review	X	X	X	X	X	X	X	X	X	X	
Project development	X										
Sending an official request for a research projcct by a primary health care provider.		X									
Research proposal summary sent to primary healthcare provider		X									
Project review by primary			X								

health care provider											
Sending ethical aspects and suggestions requested by the primary health care provider.											
Collection of information at the primary health care provider (Application of instruments)											
Information processing (Database and tabulation)											
Information analysis											
University vacations											
University reinstatement											

Final report prepared and sent to committee											
Thesis proofreading											
Approval of final report by the research committee											
Substantiation of thesis (To the primary health care provider -											

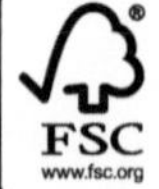

MIX
Papier aus verantwortungsvollen Quellen
Paper from responsible sources
FSC® C105338

Printed by Books on Demand GmbH, Norderstedt / Germany